Home Sweet Home:

Navigating Senior Living Options

M.A. Gorre

Contents

Introduction

Purpose of the Book

The choices surrounding senior living options are often compli-
cated and complex, filled with emotional and practical considerations. As someone who has worked for years as a nurse in long-term
care, I have witnessed firsthand the uncertainties, challenges, and
questions that elderly individuals and their families face. This book
aims to serve as a comprehensive guide that navigates you through
the various options available for senior living—aging in place, moving to an independent or assisted living community, or considering
specialized care facilities. With expert advice, real-life testimonials, and
practical tools, this guide aims to provide you and your family the
peace of mind from making well-informed decisions.

Who This Book Is For

This book is designed to be a resource for a broad audience:

    1. **Seniors**: Whether planning for your future or considering
immediate changes, this book offers insights to help you

make choices that align with your lifestyle and needs.

2. **Family Members**: Adult children, spouses, and relatives will find this book invaluable for understanding what their loved ones might require regarding comfort, care, and independence.

3. **Caregivers**: Both professional and non-professional caregivers can benefit from the detailed information and practical advice on these pages.

4. **Healthcare Professionals**: Doctors, nurses, social workers, and other healthcare providers will find this book a valuable resource to recommend to patients and their families.

How to Use This Book

The book is structured to offer a linear but flexible approach to understanding senior living options:

1. **Begin with Self-Assessment**: Chapters 2 and 11 focus on understanding the importance of choice and the need for maintaining independence and autonomy. These chapters will help you assess your or your loved one's needs.

2. **Explore Individual Options**: Chapters 3 through 7 provide an in-depth look at each living option. You can read them sequentially or focus on the opportunities that interest you the most.

3. **Compare and Contrast**: Chapter 8 is dedicated to comparing all the options to help you make an informed decision.

4. **Plan Ahead**: Chapters 9 and 12 offer advice on legal, financial, and emotional preparation for transitioning to a new living situation.

5. **Practical Tools and Resources**: Chapter 13 offers a compendium of resources, checklists, and tools to assist you in making your decision.

6. **Engage with Interactive Elements**: Throughout the book, you'll find interactive worksheets, quizzes, and checklists that help you personalize the information to your situation.

By carefully progressing through these sections and using the tools provided, you can arrive at a decision that brings comfort and a sense of certainty, knowing that you have thoroughly considered all options and their ramifications.

Understanding the Importance of Choice

♥

Emotional Well-being

When contemplating the plethora of senior living options available, emotional well-being is frequently overshadowed by practical considerations such as finances and healthcare. However, emotional health is a critical pillar impacting quality of life and physical health. Understanding its importance and how it correlates with the choice of senior living is essential for deciding that you or your loved one will be content with in the long run.

**The Role of Emotional Health in Aging

Aging is not merely a biological process but also a psychological journey. Emotional well-being can influence various health outcomes, including longevity, susceptibility to illness, and even recovery from physical ailments. A choice that aligns with an individual's emotional needs can result in a happier, more fulfilling life and, consequently, better overall health.

Emotional Autonomy

The feeling of being in control is deeply intertwined with emotional well-being. One's housing situation in senior years can significantly affect this sense of autonomy. For some, aging in place offers a sense of control and continuity, while for others, assisted living or specialized care facilities may provide a newfound freedom from the burdens of home maintenance or health-related limitations.

Social Connections

The need for social interaction doesn't wane with age; if anything, it becomes more critical. Loneliness can lead to numerous health issues, such as depression, increased stress, and cognitive decline. When choosing a living situation, consider how easy it will be to maintain and make new social connections. Independent and assisted living communities often offer built-in social activities but can also mean leaving a long-established community behind.

Staying Engaged and Purposeful

Purpose plays a significant role in emotional well-being. Whether through hobbies, community involvement, or family, having a sense of purpose can impact mental health. Consider how each living option will allow you or your loved one to engage with interests and activities that give life meaning.

Identity and Familiarity

Our homes, neighbourhoods, and communities are integral to our identity. Emotional well-being often depends on the comfort and familiarity we experience in our surroundings. This is especially important for individuals considering whether to age in place or move to an entirely new setting. Weigh how much personal identity is tied to the current living situation and what would be gained or lost by making a move.

Mental Health Support

All the senior living options should provide mental health support through professional services or a supportive community atmosphere. Ensuring that emotional needs will be met is as crucial as any other factor when choosing senior living.

Financial Considerations

Navigating the complexities of senior living options is not solely a matter of personal preference or medical needs; finances play an equally pivotal role. Financial considerations often dictate what options are accessible, feasible, and sustainable in the long term. Below are vital aspects that delve into the financial implications of choosing the right senior living.

The Cost Spectrum of Senior Living

Different living options come with additional cost structures. Aging in place may require home modifications or in-home care, which can be costly. Independent living communities typically involve a monthly fee that covers a range of services, while assisted living and nursing homes often have higher costs due to the level of care provided. It is knowing what you can afford now and in the long term.

Understanding the Hidden Costs

The apparent costs, such as rent or a mortgage, utilities, and primary healthcare, are easy to plan. However, each option may have hidden or unexpected costs. These can range from maintenance fees in an independent living community to out-of-pocket expenses for specialized medical care in a nursing home. Being financially prepared means being aware of both the obvious and the hidden costs.

Insurance, Medicare, and Medicaid

Understanding what your insurance covers and the benefits provided by Medicare and Medicaid can drastically impact your choices. While Medicare might cover certain aspects of assisted living or nursing home care, it generally does not cover long-term care. Medicaid, on the other hand, may cover long-term care but has strict eligibility requirements. Thoroughly investigate what each policy offers and how that aligns with your needs.

Estate and Financial Planning

Consider consulting a financial advisor to understand how your current estate and finances can be best organized to facilitate your preferred living situation. This could involve setting up a trust, reallocating investments, or even selling assets to free up funds.

Financial Assistance and Subsidies

Some states and organizations offer financial assistance programs for seniors. Whether it's a subsidy for home modifications to enable aging in place or financial aid for assisted living, such options can make specific paths more accessible.

Flexibility for Changing Needs

Your financial situation and healthcare needs are not static; they will change over time. Choosing an option that offers some financial flexibility can be beneficial. For instance, some independent and assisted living communities provide tiered care services you can opt into as your needs change, allowing for a smoother financial transition.

Family Contributions

It's common for family members to contribute financially to their loved ones' senior living arrangements. If this is an option in your situation, transparent, open communication is essential to ensure everyone is on the same page regarding financial commitments and expectations.

Family Dynamics

Deciding on a senior living option is seldom a solitary decision. Family plays an instrumental role in both the process and the outcome. Understanding the family dynamics can help make decisions more consensual and less fraught with conflict or regret.

The Role of Family in Decision-Making

In an ideal world, the entire family would be united in the decision-making process, offering different perspectives but ultimately working toward the same goal: the well-being of their elderly loved one. However, familial relationships can be complex, with other individuals holding different opinions, responsibilities, and emotional stakes in the decision.

Open Communication

Clear and open communication among family members is essential from the get-go. Involve all key parties in the discussions and consider holding regular family meetings to ensure everyone is updated on developments and options being considered.

Balancing Opinions and Needs

Family members may have different views on the best course of action based on their experiences, beliefs, or logistical constraints. It's essential to strike a balance between respecting everyone's opinions and focusing on the needs of the individual living in the chosen setting.

Long-Distance Family Members

In today's global society, it's common for family members to be spread across cities, states, or even countries. Remote involvement via digital platforms can be a boon, but it can also complicate decision-making. Establishing a reliable way for long-distance family members to be included in discussions and visits to potential living facilities is essential.

Caregiver Dynamics

Often, one family member assumes the primary caregiver role, which can cause tension. The primary caregiver may have insights into the daily needs and challenges other family members are not privy to. Their opinions should be weighed significantly, but this should not eclipse the collective family decision.

Children and Grandchildren

Remember that the decision also affects younger generations. Whether it's giving up a family home, relocating to a distant facility, or the emotional impact of seeing a loved one move to a more restrictive environment, the repercussions echo through the family.

Emotional Factors

Emotions run high when facing such pivotal decisions. Guilt, a sense of obligation, or a desire to repay past kindnesses can all influence family dynamics. Emotional decisions are not necessarily wrong but should be acknowledged and balanced with practical considerations.

Financial Contributions and Expectations

If family members contribute financially to the senior living arrangement, this may give them more say in the decision. Such dynamics need to be managed carefully to avoid conflict.

Overall Conclusion

Choosing the right senior living option is multifaceted beyond the surface-level considerations of healthcare needs and practicalities. It requires a nuanced understanding of the individual's emotional well-being, the complexities of family dynamics, and the suitability of financial constraints.

Emotional well-being is an abstract concept and a critical pillar influencing quality of life and overall health. Neglecting to factor in emotional needs could result in a choice that fails to bring happiness, fulfillment, and general well-being. Similarly, family plays an invaluable role in decision-making, offering both support and complexity. Open communication and empathy are essential in navigating the range of family opinions and needs, leading to a choice that respects everyone involved.

Lastly, understanding the financial dimensions of each senior living option can mean the difference between peace of mind and an unanticipated struggle. Being aware of the hidden costs and insurance benefits allows for a sustainable choice that won't jeopardize financial security.

Combining these three essential elements—emotional well-being, family dynamics, and financial considerations—you can make an informed, balanced decision that meets immediate needs and stands the test of time. This comprehensive approach ensures that the choice made genuinely feels like home, respects the needs and wishes of the individual, and garners the support of the family, all while maintaining financial health.

Aging in Place

♥

What Does it Mean?

The term "Aging in Place" refers to the ability of an individual to reside within their community securely, self-sufficiently, and with ease, irrespective of age, financial status, or level of capability

It is a concept that resonates deeply with many people because it taps into the desire for familiarity, autonomy, and the preservation of a well-loved living space.

Autonomy and Freedom

Aging in place is often equated with a sense of autonomy and freedom. It allows the individual to make choices about their daily life, routines, and healthcare, all within the comfort of their home. The notion of control that comes with living in a familiar environment can significantly impact emotional well-being.

Continuity and Familiarity

Our homes are often filled with memories and associations that make them irreplaceable. Being able to age in place means maintaining a sense of continuity in one's life. It allows individuals to stay connected to their community, neighbours, and, often, nearby family members.

Customization of Needs

Adapting the home environment to fit changing needs when aging in place is possible. This can include installing grab bars in the bathroom, adding a stairlift, or making the home wheelchair-accessible. The customization allows the individual to address their specific needs and medical conditions.

Financial Aspects

Contrary to what some might assume, aging in place doesn't always translate to financial savings. While it may eliminate the need to pay for an assisted living facility or a nursing home, there could be considerable costs involved in home modifications, ongoing maintenance, and in-home care services. Thorough financial planning is vital to ensure sustainability.

Family Involvement

The choice to age in place often involves the family's support, both emotionally and logistically. Family members may take turns visiting, assisting with chores, and providing companionship. The closeness to family can be both a boon and a challenge, depending on family dynamics.

Healthcare Considerations

One of the main challenges of aging in place is managing healthcare needs. While in-home healthcare services are available, they may not offer the extensive medical facilities that a specialized institution can provide. Being realistic about healthcare needs is crucial when deciding to age in place.

Safety Concerns

Safety is a significant factor, especially for those who live alone. Emergency alert systems, regular check-ins from family or healthcare providers, and a well-maintained home can mitigate safety risks.

Psychological Benefits

A sense of ownership and an emotional attachment to one's home can have significant psychological benefits. These dynamic aspects are invaluable and can positively affect mental health, reinforcing the desire to age in place.

Pros and Cons

Ageing in place is a deeply personal decision influenced by various factors, including emotional ties, healthcare needs, family dynamics, and financial considerations. Below are some pros and cons that can provide further insight into what aging in place entails.

Pros

1. **Emotional Comfort**: Staying in a familiar environment can be emotionally comforting and provide a sense of continuity. Homes often hold cherished memories, making them irreplaceable.

2. **Personal Freedom**: Aging in place offers the autonomy to live according to one's preferences, from meal timings to daily activities, which can significantly contribute to overall well-being.

3. **Customization**: The home can be modified to suit the individual's specific needs, whether installing grab bars in the bathroom or ramps for wheelchair access.

4. **Family and Community Ties**: Maintaining long-standing relationships and community connections can offer emotional support and reduce feelings of isolation.

5. **Potential Cost Savings**: Depending on healthcare needs and the extent of home modifications required, aging in place can be more cost-effective in some cases than institutional care.

6. **Pet Ownership**: For many, the ability to keep pets is a significant advantage that contributes to emotional well-being.

Cons

1. **Safety Risks**: As one age, the risk of falls or medical emergencies at home increases. Without immediate professional care, these situations can escalate.

2. **Maintenance Challenges**: Homeownership is responsible for upkeep, which can become physically and financially challenging.

3. **Limited Healthcare**: Even with home health services, the level of medical care may be less comprehensive than what's available in a specialized facility.

4. **Social Isolation**: Living alone can sometimes result in feelings of loneliness or depression, mainly if family and friends are not nearby.

5. **Financial Strain**: The cost of retrofitting a home to suit changing needs and hiring in-home care can quickly add up, causing financial stress.

6. **Complex Family Dynamics**: Family members may have strong opinions about aging in place, and their ability to contribute to care can vary, leading to possible conflicts.

Home Modifications for Safety and Comfort

One of the most significant aspects of successfully aging in place is modifying the home to meet evolving physical needs and safety concerns. Here, we delve into various changes that can be made to create a home environment that is both comfortable and secure.

Entry and Exit Points

1. **Ramps**: Replace steps with ramps for easier access, mainly if wheelchairs or walkers are used.

2. **Handrails**: Install sturdy bars on both sides of staircases and ramps.

3. **Keyless Entry**: Consider adding a keyless entry system to eliminate the need to fumble with keys.

Living Areas

1. **Open Floor Plan**: Open spaces for more effortless movement, mainly if mobility devices are used.

2. **Non-slip Flooring**: Replace slippery floors with non-slip options to reduce the risk of falls.

3. **Furniture Arrangement**: Ensure furniture does not obstruct walkways and is sturdy enough to assist in getting up.

Kitchen

1. **Lower Countertops**: Lowering countertops and sinks can make kitchen tasks easier for those who are seated.

2. **Pull-out Shelves**: Use pull-out shelves in cabinets for easier access.

3. **Levers Over Knobs**: Opt for lever-style faucet handles in-

stead of knobs.

Bathrooms

1. **Walk-in Showers**: Replace bathtubs with walk-in showers with a minimal step-over threshold.

2. **Grab Bars**: Install grab bars near the toilet and in the shower or tub area.

3. **Raised Toilet Seats**: Consider a higher toilet seat or an adjustable seat for easier sitting and standing.

Bedrooms

1. **Bed Rails**: Install bed rails to assist in getting in and out of bed.

2. **Closet Organizers**: Use pull-down or adjustable closet rods for easier access to clothes.

3. **Ample Lighting**: Ensure there's sufficient lighting to move around safely.

General Home Features

1. **Lighting**: Improve lighting throughout the house to avoid shadows and dark spots that could lead to falls.

2. **Emergency Systems**: Install a reliable medical alert system.

3. **Smoke and Carbon Monoxide Detectors**: Ensure detectors are working and are easily accessible.

Financial Considerations

Making home modifications can be costly. Some may be covered by insurance or grants for seniors, but most will be out-of-pocket expenses. Budgeting for these changes is crucial when planning to age in place.

Technology to Assist in Aging in Place

As the world becomes increasingly digitized, technology is pivotal in facilitating aging. With advancements in smart home devices, telemedicine, and other technological tools, seniors can experience excellent safety, convenience, and health monitoring while maintaining independence.

Health Monitoring Devices

1. **Wearable Fitness Trackers**: These devices can monitor basic health metrics like heart rate, sleep quality, and activity level.

2. **Telemedicine Platforms**: Allow seniors to consult with healthcare providers from the comfort of their own homes.

3. **Medication Dispensers**: Automatic dispensers can be programmed to release medications at specific times, reducing the chance of missing a dose.

Communication Tools

1. **Video Calling**: Applications like Zoom or Skype allow maintaining face-to-face contact with family and friends.

2. **Voice-activated Assistants**: Devices like Amazon's Alexa or Google Home can help seniors send messages, make calls, or perform internet searches through voice commands.

Home Safety

1. **Smart Doorbells and Locks**: These provide added security by allowing homeowners to see who is at their door without opening it.

2. **Fall Detection Systems**: Some wearable devices come equipped with fall detection, sending an alert to designated contacts in the event of a fall.

3. **Bright Smoke and Carbon Monoxide Detectors**: These devices can send alerts to your phone, providing an additional layer of safety.

Convenience and Comfort

1. **Smart Thermostats**: Allow for remote adjustment of home temperature.

2. **Voice-activated Lights and Appliances** Can be controlled

via voice commands or programmed to function at specific times.

3. **Grocery Delivery Apps**: Eliminate the need to go to the store, making it easier for those with mobility issues.

Staying Active and Engaged

1. **Online Learning Platforms**: Offer courses and tutorials to keep the mind active.

2. **Streaming Services**: Provide endless entertainment options for seniors, from movies to exercise classes.

Financial Considerations

While technology can significantly assist in aging in place, a cost factor is involved. It is essential to budget for these technologies and research whether governmental or organizational grants can subsidize them.

Cost Analysis

Deciding to age in place involves careful financial planning. While there may be emotional and practical advantages to staying in your home, the costs can add up. This section aims to break down these costs to aid in making a more informed decision.

Home Modifications

1. **Ramps and Railings**: Costs can vary significantly based on the materials and complexity, ranging from a few hundred to several thousand dollars.

2. **Bathroom Modifications**: Walk-in showers, grab bars, and raised toilets can cost anywhere from $500 to $10,000, depending on the extent of the changes.

3. **Kitchen Adjustments**: Lowering countertops and installing pull-out shelves can range from $1,000 to $20,000.

Technology

1. **Smart Home Devices**: Expect to spend at least $200 to $1,000 on smart thermostats, doorbells, and locks.

2. **Health Monitoring Devices**: Wearables and medication dispensers can range from $50 to $500.

3. **Subscription Services**: Some technologies come with ongoing subscription fees, which can add up over time.

In-Home Care

1. **Non-Medical In-home Care**: Costs average around $20 to $30 per hour, but this can vary based on location and the level of service needed.

2. **Skilled Nursing**: The cost can skyrocket to $40 to $100 per hour if specialized care is required.

Maintenance and Utilities

1. **General Maintenance**: The annual cost of maintaining a home can be 1% to 3% of the home's value.

2. **Utilities**: Consider the ongoing costs of electricity, heating, and cooling, which vary greatly depending on the home and location.

Insurance and Taxes

1. **Home Insurance**: Premiums may increase if the home undergoes significant modifications.

2. **Property Taxes**: These are an ongoing expense that can rise over time.

Additional Costs

1. **Transportation**: If driving is no longer an option, budget for public transportation or rideshare services.

2. **Groceries and Supplies**: Include the cost of grocery delivery services if applicable.

Funding and Financial Assistance

1. **Reverse Mortgages**: This option allows homeowners to

convert part of their home equity into cash.

2. **Grants and Subsidies**: Some government programs can help cover the costs of home modifications.

3. **Long-term Care Insurance**: Check if your policy covers any aging costs in place.

Final Conclusion

Aging in place is a deeply personal and multifaceted decision that extends far beyond the simple comfort of familiarity. It encompasses emotional well-being, healthcare needs, family dynamics, technological advancements, and financial considerations. The desire to maintain independence and the comfort of a well-known environment often needs to be balanced against practical aspects like safety and cost.

The evolution of technology is a remarkable asset in this context, offering a range of solutions that empower seniors to control their health, safety, and daily activities. When integrated thoughtfully, these technologies can significantly contribute to the quality of life and overall well-being.

Simultaneously, home modifications are essential, not merely for convenience but as crucial investments in long-term safety and quality of life. While some of these modifications may seem minor or even luxurious, they can dramatically affect the feasibility of aging in place and an individual's ability to live independently.

Financial considerations are equally imperative. With various hidden and obvious costs involved, planning for the economic aspect is vital to ensure you or your loved one can age in place without compromising financial health. These costs should be weighed against other senior living options to assess which is the most financially feasible over the long term.

Finally, the emotional aspects and family dynamics should never be overlooked. These are often the linchpin in the decision-making process. Open, empathetic communication among all parties involved can pave the way for a choice that meets the needs and enriches the life of the individual, as well as their family.

In summary, the decision to age in place is complex and multi-dimensional. It requires thorough analysis, covering emotional, financial, healthcare, and familial factors. By taking a holistic approach, you can arrive at a well-informed decision that not only meets basic needs but also contributes to a fulfilling and secure life during the later years

Independent Living Communities

Overview

Independent Living Communities offer an excellent middle ground for seniors looking for a blend of independence and convenience. These communities provide private living spaces, often in apartments or tiny homes. They are designed to remove some of the burdens of home maintenance and upkeep, offering residents more freedom to enjoy their later years.

What Independent Living Communities Offer

1. **Community Atmosphere**: One of the primary benefits is the community setting, which allows for social interaction, communal activities, and a sense of belonging.

2. **Facilities and Amenities**: These include fitness centers,

swimming pools, communal dining areas, and sometimes onsite healthcare services.

3. **Safety and Security**: With security personnel and emergency response systems, these communities provide an added layer of protection.

4. **Transportation Services**: Many communities offer shuttle services to nearby shopping centers, medical appointments, and community events.

5. **Maintenance-Free Living**: The community staff typically handles lawn care, housekeeping, and repairs.

Financial Considerations

1. **Entrance Fees**: Some communities require a significant upfront fee, followed by monthly charges.

2. **Monthly Expenses** vary widely depending on location, services, and amenities.

3. **Additional Costs**: Additional services, like specialized healthcare or premium amenities, may cost extra.

Emotional and Lifestyle Aspects

1. **Freedom and Independence**: These communities offer more independence than other senior living options like assisted living or nursing homes.

2. **Social Opportunities**: The built-in community aspect provides numerous opportunities for socialization, thereby combating feelings of loneliness and isolation that some seniors experience.

3. **Limited Healthcare**: While some communities offer essential healthcare services, they are generally not equipped to deal with more severe health issues.

Pros and Cons

The decision to move into an Independent Living Community is often nuanced, influenced by various factors ranging from financial capability to social needs. Below, we explore some of this living arrangement's most common advantages and disadvantages.

Pros

1. **Socialization**: One of the most significant advantages is the community atmosphere. Regularly scheduled activities, clubs, and communal spaces make it easier to forge new friendships and maintain an active social life.

2. **Reduced Maintenance**: Say goodbye to lawn mowing, plumbing repairs, or snow shovelling. The community typically handles these, allowing residents to focus on more enjoyable activities.

3. **Safety and Security**: These communities often have 24-hour security, emergency response systems, and some-

times even healthcare staff, providing peace of mind to residents and their families.

4. **Amenities**: Residents usually have access to various amenities such as fitness centers, swimming pools, libraries, and sometimes even on-site dining options, enhancing the quality of life.

5. **Transportation**: Many Independent Living Communities offer shuttle services to grocery stores, medical appointments, and community events, reducing the need for a personal vehicle.

Cons

1. **Cost**: While they offer many amenities and services, these communities can be expensive. Monthly fees and additional charges can add up quickly, requiring a stable financial plan.

2. **Limited Medical Care**: While some offer essential healthcare services, they are not substitutes for skilled nursing facilities or other types of intensive medical care.

3. **Less Personal Space**: Generally, the living spaces in these communities are smaller than a typical home, which may require downsizing possessions.

4. **Regulated Environment**: While these communities offer independence, they come with rules and guidelines that residents must follow, which might not suit everyone.

5. **Lack of Personalization**: Because the community typically

takes care of maintenance and landscaping, there may be restrictions on how much you can personalize your living space.

Activities and Amenities

One of the main attractions of Independent Living Communities is the vast array of activities and amenities available to residents. These extras can significantly contribute to an individual's quality of life, offering leisure and opportunities for personal growth, physical fitness, and social interaction. Here's a breakdown:

Activities

1. **Social Gatherings** could include everything from movie nights and barbecues to book clubs and game nights.

2. **Fitness Classes**: Many communities offer various fitness classes, like yoga, Pilates, and water aerobics, tailored to a senior audience.

3. **Educational Programs**: Some communities partner with local colleges or experts to offer lectures, workshops, or accredited courses.

4. **Cultural Events**: Outings to museums, theatres, or concerts can be a part of the community's social calendar as an in-house performance.

5. **Skill-Building**: Cooking classes, computer courses, or language learning are also popular activities that communities

may offer.

Amenities

1. **Fitness Centers**: Modern gym facilities often tailored to the needs of seniors.

2. **Swimming Pools**: Many communities offer indoor or outdoor pools, sometimes with lifeguards and instructors.

3. **Dining Facilities**: Some have communal dining halls with meal plans, while others offer private dining options.

4. **Libraries and Media Rooms**: Quiet spaces can be available for reading or access to computers and the Internet.

5. **Health and Wellness Centers**: While not a substitute for full-fledged medical facilities, these can offer essential healthcare services.

6. **Transportation**: Shuttle services for shopping, medical appointments, and community events are commonly provided.

Cost Analysis

Understanding the cost structure of Independent Living Communities is crucial for making an informed decision. The costs can be multifaceted, involving upfront payments and ongoing monthly fees, among other potential charges. Here's a breakdown to help you navigate these financial waters:

Initial Costs

1. **Entrance Fees**: Some communities require an upfront entrance fee, which can range from a few thousand to several hundred thousand dollars, depending on the community's policies and the services they offer.

2. **Security Deposits**: In addition to or instead of an entrance fee, a refundable or non-refundable security deposit might be required.

Ongoing Costs

1. **Monthly Fees**: These usually cover essential services like rent, utilities, maintenance, and some communal amenities. Fees can range from $1,500 to $6,000 monthly, depending on location, room size, and included amenities.

2. **Meal Plans**: Some communities offer optional meal plans for an additional fee.

3. **Activity Fees**: The monthly fee might not cover special activities or excursions and could entail extra charges.

4. **Healthcare Services**: Some communities offer essential healthcare services for an additional fee, but these are generally not comprehensive.

Additional Costs

1. **Laundry and Housekeeping**: While some communities include these services in the monthly fee, others charge extra.

2. **Parking**: If you have a vehicle, there may be an additional monthly parking fee.

3. **Pet Fees**: If the community is pet-friendly, expect to pay a pet deposit and possibly a monthly pet fee.

4. **Upgrades**: Specialized amenities, like a larger apartment or a better view, could also come at a premium.

Financial Aid and Discounts

1. **Veteran's Benefits**: Some communities offer discounts for veterans.

2. **Medicaid**: In some cases, Medicaid may cover part of the costs, although this is rare for Independent Living Communities.

3. **Long-Term Care Insurance**: If you have a policy, check to see if it covers any of the costs associated with independent living.

Independent Living Communities offer a valuable option for seniors who cherish their independence but seek to minimize home maintenance responsibilities. There may be an additional monthly parking fee if you have a vehicle and desire increased social opportunities. These communities come with a range of amenities and activities designed to enrich residents' lives physically, intellectually, and socially. However, it's essential to consider that these features might come with additional costs or may be included in the monthly fees. Individuals and families should take a comprehensive approach when exploring this option, factoring in the visible upfront costs and various potential hidden or future expenses. Consulting a financial advisor to create a detailed budget can be invaluable for making an informed decision that aligns with lifestyle preferences and financial capabilities. While Independent Living Communities offer many benefits, they are not a one-size-fits-all solution and should be evaluated carefully to ensure they meet individual needs, lifestyle goals, and financial constraints.

Nursing Homes

♥

When is it Necessary?

Determining the right time to move to a nursing home can be emotionally fraught, but sometimes, it's the best or only feasible option. The decision typically depends on several factors:

Medical Needs

1. **Chronic Illness**: Conditions like Alzheimer's, dementia, or other cognitive decline often require specialized care that cannot be provided at home or in less equipped senior living communities.

2. **Intensive Medical Care**: Some seniors may require round-the-clock medical monitoring, frequent medication adjustments, or regular treatments like dialysis that can only be efficiently provided in a nursing home.

3. **Mobility Issues**: Severe mobility challenges, like bedridden

or requiring assistance for all movements, may make nursing home care necessary.

Caregiver Strain

1. **Availability**: Family members might be unable to provide the care needed due to work commitments, distance, or health issues.

2. **Expertise**: Even when family members are available, they may lack the specialized skills required for particular medical conditions.

3. **Emotional Toll**: The stress of constant caregiving can affect the well-being of family caregivers, which may necessitate a move to a more supportive environment.

Safety Concerns

1. **Frequent Falls**: If a senior is experiencing regular falls or accidents, a nursing home can provide a more controlled environment with professional oversight.

2. **Wandering**: Some seniors, especially those with cognitive decline, might walk and expose themselves to risks that can only be mitigated in a secure facility.

Quality of Life

1. **Social Interaction**: If the senior is isolated and lacks social interaction, a nursing home can provide a community setting.

2. **Comprehensive Care**: Nursing homes offer multidimensional medical, nutritional, and psychological care that can significantly improve a senior's quality of life.

Pros and Cons

Choosing a nursing home for oneself or a loved one is a decision fraught with emotional, financial, and practical implications. Therefore, understanding the advantages and drawbacks is essential for making an informed choice.

Pros

1. **24/7 Medical Care**: One of the most significant benefits of nursing homes is the continuous access to medical care and monitoring.

2. **Skilled Staff**: These facilities employ trained healthcare professionals like nurses, physical therapists, and occupational therapists, offering various medical services.

3. **Structured Environment**: The regimented schedule for meals, medication, and activities can provide comfort and routine, especially for seniors with cognitive impairments.

4. **Social Opportunities**: Despite losing some independence, nursing homes offer social interaction that seniors might not

get if they lived alone or with busy family members.

5. **All-Inclusive**: Generally, the cost covers room, board, and most healthcare services, eliminating the worry of handling multiple bills.

6. **Nutritional Management**: With dietitians on staff, nursing homes can cater to various dietary needs and restrictions, ensuring balanced nutrition.

7. **Safety**: Nursing homes are equipped with safety measures like emergency call buttons, handrails, and secure entrances to ensure the well-being of residents.

Cons

1. **Cost**: Nursing homes can be prohibitively expensive, often requiring a significant out-of-pocket contribution even with insurance.

2. **Loss of Independence**: Residents often have to adapt to a schedule and may have limited personal space, impacting their sense of autonomy.

3. **Emotional Impact**: The move can be emotionally challenging for the resident and their family, sometimes causing feelings of abandonment or guilt.

4. **Limited Privacy**: Shared rooms are standard, which can be uncomfortable for those used to living alone.

5. **Quality Variance**: The standard of care can vary signifi-

cantly between facilities, making the selection process crucial but challenging.

6. **Institutional Atmosphere**: Despite efforts to make these facilities homely, some may feel impersonal and institutional, affecting the resident's morale.

7. **Regulations and Rules**: There can be numerous rules and regulations that residents must follow, which might feel restrictive.

Financial Aspects

When selecting a nursing home, understanding the financial implications is crucial for making an informed decision. Costs can be significant and often catch families unprepared. Here's a breakdown of what you need to consider:

Types of Costs

1. **Admission Fees**: Many nursing homes have an initial admission fee, which may or may not be refundable.

2. **Monthly Charges**: The bulk of the expense is typically the monthly fee, which covers room, board, and primary medical care.

3. **Additional Services**: Specialized therapies, personal care items, and certain medications might incur additional costs.

4. **Laundry and Housekeeping**: While some nursing homes

include this in the basic package, others might charge extra.

Payment Options

1. **Private Pay**: Many people pay for nursing homes out-of-pocket, at least initially. This method is straightforward but can be financially draining.

2. **Medicare** covers particular nursing home stays but has strict eligibility criteria, often requiring a prior hospital stay and usually covering only short-term stays.

3. **Medicaid**: If you qualify, Medicaid can help cover long-term nursing home costs, but eligibility rules and coverage can vary by state.

4. **Long-term Care Insurance**: If purchased in advance, these policies can cover a significant portion of nursing home costs.

5. **Veteran's Benefits**: Some seniors may be eligible for the Department of Veterans Affairs aid.

Financial Planning

1. **Consult a Financial Advisor**: Given the complexity, consulting a financial advisor knowledgeable in elder care can provide invaluable insights.

2. **Cost Projection**: A detailed financial plan should be made for future cost increases due to inflation or changes in

healthcare needs.

3. **Asset Management**: Managing assets strategically can sometimes help qualify for Medicaid or other assistance programs.

Final Conclusion

Choosing a nursing home is a multifaceted decision that demands careful consideration of emotional, financial, and healthcare needs. The need for a nursing home arises when other options, such as home care or assisted living, become inadequate due to escalating medical requirements, caregiver limitations, or safety concerns. While nursing homes deliver an invaluable service of round-the-clock medical care for those with complex health needs, they also have substantial emotional and lifestyle implications.

Understanding the financial dimensions is crucial for comprehensive planning. Costs can be daunting, and not just the obvious ones. Additional expenses for specialized therapies, personal care, and medications can increase. Various payment options, including Medicare, Medicaid, long-term care insurance, and out-of-pocket payments, offer different pros and cons that must be weighed carefully. Because of the complexity and significant financial implications, consulting a financial advisor specialized in elder care can be immensely helpful.

Given the considerable emotional, financial, and lifestyle factors involved, this decision should ideally be collaborative, involving the senior—if possible—along with family members and healthcare providers. It's a choice that affects the lives of the old involved and those who care for them. As such, it's essential to weigh all these aspects thoughtfully to make the best decision for everyone involved.

Specialized Care Facilities

Memory Care Units

Overview

Memory Care Units are specialized residential facilities designed to meet the unique needs of individuals with Alzheimer's, dementia, and other memory-related conditions. Unlike traditional nursing homes, these units are tailored to provide a safe environment and specialized care to manage symptoms, maximize quality of life, and slow the progression of cognitive decline.

When Is It Necessary?

Memory Care Units become a necessary option when an individual's cognitive impairments reach a point where they require specialized attention and care that cannot be provided in a standard senior living facility or at home. Signs include severe memory loss, frequent wandering, aggressive behaviours, and increased medical needs that regular assisted living or nursing home staff cannot handle.

Pros and Cons

Pros:

1. **Focused Care:** The staff is specially trained in dementia care.

2. **Security:** Enhanced safety measures to prevent wandering and self-harm.

3. **Structured Environment:** Customized activities and therapies to improve cognitive and physical function.

4. **Family Support:** Support groups and counselling services for family members.

Cons:

1. **High Costs:** Specialized services and high staff-to-resident ratios drive up costs.

2. **Limited Independence:** Personal freedom is restricted due to cognitive decline and safety measures.

3. **Emotional Toll:** It can be emotionally challenging for families to transition a loved one to a specialized facility.

Financial Aspects

Memory Care Units are often more expensive than other residential care options, with costs ranging significantly depending on location, level of care, and amenities. While some expenses may be covered by private insurance or Medicaid, Medicare generally does not cover long-term stays in these specialized units. Families may also explore other financial support options, such as Veterans' benefits or grants for dementia care.

Rehabilitation Centers

Overview

Rehabilitation Centers provide specialized care and treatment to individuals recovering from surgery, injury, or illness. Unlike standard nursing homes, these facilities focus on short-term, intensive therapeutic interventions to restore an individual's independence and return them to their original state of health, or as close to it as possible.

When Is It Necessary?

Rehabilitation centers are often recommended following hospital discharge for conditions that require concentrated therapeutic efforts. This could range from stroke recovery to orthopedic surgeries like knee or hip replacements. The objective is to offer intense, multidisciplinary therapies, including physical, occupational, and speech therapies that you can't efficiently receive at home or in an outpatient setting.

Pros and Cons

Pros:

1. **Specialized Care:** Highly trained professionals focus on specific recovery goals.

2. **Structured Environment:** Daily routines of therapies and medical check-ups ensure optimal recovery.

3. **Advanced Equipment:** Access to specialized equipment not available in home settings.

4. **Transitioning Care:** Acts as an intermediate step between hospital and home, aiding in adjustment.

Cons:

1. **Limited Personal Freedom:** Highly scheduled days may offer little personal time.

2. **Cost:** Private insurance may cover a portion, but out-of-pocket expenses can be high.

3. **Limited Stay:** Typically not designed for long-term care.

Hospice Care

Overview

Hospice Care is a specialized form of medical and emotional support focused on providing comfort and quality of life for individuals in the late stages of a terminal illness. The care is not aimed at curing the disease but rather at managing symptoms and providing emotional and spiritual support for the individual and their family.

When Is It Necessary?

Hospice care is generally recommended when curative treatment is no longer effective or desired, and the individual is expected to have six months or less to live. The focus is on palliative care—relieving pain and other distressing symptoms—while providing psychological, social, and spiritual support.

Pros and Cons

Pros:

1. **Holistic Care:** Provides medical, emotional, and spiritual support.

2. **Family Involvement:** Encourages the family to participate in the care and decision-making.

3. **Comfort-Oriented:** Focuses on patient comfort and quality of life.

4. **Multi-Disciplinary Team:** Involves a team of healthcare providers, including doctors, nurses, social workers, and chaplains.

Cons:

1. **End-of-Life Focus:** Some individuals and family members find it emotionally challenging to shift focus from cure to comfort.

2. **Home-Based Challenges:** While hospice can be provided at home, this can be emotionally and physically draining for family caregivers.

3. **Cost:** Medicare often covers hospice, but not all services may be covered, and private insurance varies widely.

Financial Aspects

While Medicare and most private insurance cover hospice care, it's crucial to clarify what is and isn't included. Out-of-pocket expenses can arise for non-covered services or medications. Always consult with your insurance provider and the hospice organization to understand your financial responsibilities fully.

Final Conclusion

Choosing the appropriate form of senior care—Hospice Care, a Rehabilitation Center, or a Memory Care Unit—requires open communication, careful consideration, and a thorough understanding of various factors.

Hospice Care is a compassionate option focusing on dignity and quality of life during the end-of-life journey. While emotionally and spiritually supportive, it demands a shift from seeking a cure to providing comfort, a transition that may be challenging for the patient and their loved ones. Understanding the financial coverage is also vital to avoid unexpected costs.

Rehabilitation Centers offer specialized therapies to help individuals recover from surgeries, accidents, or illnesses. They can be cost-intensive depending on the required treatments and length of stay. Knowing what your insurance covers and understanding Medicare guidelines is crucial for budgeting and planning.

Memory Care Units provide a specialized, secure environment for individuals with memory-related conditions. While these units offer peace of mind and expert care, they often come at a higher financial cost and emotional toll on the family. Therefore, a thorough evaluation of needs, benefits, and limitations is critical for making an informed decision.

Navigating these diverse senior care options is never a one-size-fits-all situation. It is a profoundly personal, family-oriented decision requiring a holistic approach considering emotional well-being, healthcare needs, and financial capacities. Only through a well-rounded understanding of these various aspects can families arrive at a decision that truly serves the best interests of their loved ones.

Comparing Options: At a Glance

Deciding where to spend your golden years—or helping a loved one decide—can be overwhelming due to the array of options available. Below is a concise comparison of four significant senior living alternatives: Aging in Place, Independent Living Communities, Assisted Living Facilities, and Nursing Homes. This overview aims to provide a quick snapshot to help you understand the main differences and guide you toward a decision that best aligns with your needs.

Aging in Place

- **Suitability**: Ideal for those in good health and wishing to stay home.

- **Level of Care**: Minimal to moderate, depending on the individual's health.

- **Financial Cost**: Varies widely, depending on the need for home modifications or in-home care.

- **Lifestyle**: High level of independence, but potentially less social interaction unless proactive.

Independent Living Communities

- **Suitability**: Best for primarily independent seniors who wish to be free from home maintenance.

- **Level of Care**: Minimal; no healthcare services provided as a rule.

- **Financial Cost**: Monthly or annual fees, plus potential additional costs for extra amenities.

- **Lifestyle**: Community-based social activities are available, and amenities like gyms or pools are often included.

Assisted Living Facilities

- **Suitability**: Good for those who require assistance with daily activities but don't need complex medical care.

- **Level of Care**: Moderate; assistance with daily activities and essential medical monitoring.

- **Financial Cost**: Typically more expensive than Independent Living but less than Nursing Homes.

- **Lifestyle**: Semi-independent, organized activities, meals provided.

Nursing Homes

- **Suitability**: Designed for individuals with significant healthcare needs, including 24/7 monitoring.

- **Level of Care**: High; a full range of healthcare services, including skilled nursing.

- **Financial Cost**: Most expensive, often requiring insurance or Medicaid to offset costs.

- **Lifestyle**: Limited independence, heavily healthcare-focused.

What to Consider When Making a Choice

Selecting the most appropriate living arrangement for yourself or a loved one during the golden years is a multifaceted decision that involves several variables. Below are vital factors you should consider when making this critical choice:

Emotional Well-being

- Is the individual excited or comfortable about the prospective setting?

- Does the option align with the person's values, desires, and lifestyle?

Level of Independence

- How much daily assistance does the individual need?

- Does the person want to maintain their current lifestyle, or are they open to a change?

Health and Medical Needs

- Are specialized medical services or routine healthcare required?

- Is there a progressive health condition that will necessitate escalating care?

Financial Considerations

- What is the cost structure of each option—entry fees, monthly fees, additional costs?

- Have you consulted a financial advisor to understand how this move will impact the individual's or family's financial situation?

Social Aspects

- Does the individual enjoy solitude or prefer an active, social environment?

- Are there enough opportunities for social engagement in the considered setting?

Safety and Accessibility

- Are modifications required to make the home or facility safe and accessible?

- What is the emergency response time, and are medical facilities easily accessible?

Location

- Is it essential for the individual to stay close to family and friends?

- What is the proximity to shopping centers, healthcare facilities, and recreational activities?

Quality of Life

- What are the reviews or ratings of the facility, if applicable?

- Have you visited the site to assess the staff, amenities, and overall environment?

Family Dynamics

- Are all key family members in agreement on the best choice?

- Is the choice practical for family visits and involvement in the individual's life?

Future Needs

- Is this choice adaptable to future healthcare or lifestyle needs?

- What is the policy for transitions to higher levels of care, if needed?

By examining these factors in detail, you will be better equipped to make an informed decision that suits the individual's unique situation while considering the broader impact on family and financials. Each consideration can be like a piece of a puzzle that, when completed, reveals the most fitting living situation. Take your time to evaluate each aspect to make the best decision possible.

Legal and Financial Planning: Estate Planning

♥

E state planning is not just for the wealthy; it is a crucial aspect of preparing for the future that everyone, especially seniors, should consider. Understanding your estate can be immensely helpful if you are considering aging in place, moving to an assisted living facility, or any other living option.

Importance of Estate Planning

Planning your estate provides a structured way to distribute your assets according to your wishes after your passing. It is also a way to ensure that your medical and financial affairs are handled appropriately if you can no longer do so yourself. A well-structured estate plan can prevent family disagreements, minimize tax liability, and give you peace of mind.

Core Components

1. Last will: Your will is the cornerstone of your estate plan, outlining how your assets will be distributed and who will care for any minor children.

2. **Durable Power of Attorney**: This document appoints someone to act on your behalf in financial and legal matters if you are incapacitated.

3. **Healthcare Proxy**: Also known as a healthcare power of attorney, this designates someone to make medical decisions for you if you cannot do so.

4. **Living Will**: This outlines your preferences for life-sustaining treatments if you cannot communicate your wishes.

5. **Trusts**: These are used to manage and distribute assets, often allowing for a smoother transition and tax benefits.

6. **Beneficiary Designations**: Assets like retirement accounts and life insurance policies typically bypass your will and go directly to the beneficiaries named on these accounts.

Navigating Complexities

- **Tax Planning**: An estate plan can help minimize the tax burden on your heirs.

- **Elder Law Considerations**: As you age, you may encounter legal issues unique to seniors, such as those related to Medicare, Medicaid, and long-term care planning. An elder law attorney can be beneficial in these cases.

Involving Family and Professionals

Involving family members in your estate planning process is advisable, ensuring transparency and fewer disputes later. Furthermore, consulting with legal and financial professionals ensures that your estate plan complies with the law and meets all your needs.

Financial Planning for Senior Living

Understanding your estate can also help you make informed decisions about senior living options. For example, the sale of a home might be used to finance assisted living, or specific assets might be liquidated to provide a financial cushion for in-home care.

Power of Attorney

Introduction

Power of Attorney (POA) is often misunderstood but critical in legal and financial planning, especially for seniors contemplating various living options. It gives a designated individual the legal authority to decide on your behalf if you cannot, bill payment tasks,

Types of Power of Attorney

1. **General Power of Attorney**: This grants broad powers to the designated individual to act in various matters, including legal and financial issues.

2. **Unique or Limited Power of Attorney**: Grants authority to handle specific tasks or decisions, often for a limited time or under particular circumstances.

3. **Durable Power of Attorney**: Unlike other types, this remains in effect even if you become incapacitated, making it highly relevant for eldercare planning.

4. **Healthcare Power of Attorney**: Specifically focused on healthcare decisions should you become unable to make them yourself.

Importance in Senior Care

Whether you're aging in place or moving to a specialized care facility, a POA is essential. It ensures that someone can manage your affairs, from paying bills to making healthcare decisions, in case you cannot do so.

How to Choose an Agent

- **Trustworthiness**: The individual should be trustworthy and capable of making decisions that align with your wishes.

- **Availability**: Ensure the person is readily available to execute their duties, preferably someone who lives nearby or can travel quickly.

- **Expertise**: Choose someone who understands financial matters and legal implications or is willing to consult experts.

Implementing a Power of Attorney

- **Consult a Legal Expert**: To draft a POA, consult a legal expert to ensure it complies with state laws and addresses all necessary areas.

- **Discuss with Family**: Transparency is crucial. Discuss your decision to designate a POA with close family members to avoid misunderstandings later.

- **Record Keeping**: Make sure multiple copies of the POA are available and relevant parties, such as your healthcare provider or financial advisor, can access it.

Considerations for Different Living Options

- **Aging in Place**: A POA can handle home maintenance and bill payment tasks and necessary medical decisions.

- **Assisted Living/Nursing Homes**: A POA can assist with administrative processes and make medical decisions if needed.

- **Memory Care Units**: For those with cognitive issues, a durable POA is especially crucial for making both financial and healthcare decisions.

Conclusion

Power of Attorney and Estate Planning are critical components of comprehensive legal and financial planning for your senior years. A well-executed Power of Attorney ensures that responsible decisions are made on your behalf when you cannot do so, offering a safety net for various aspects of life, from healthcare to finances. On the other hand, effective estate planning safeguards your assets and guarantees they are distributed according to your wishes while contributing to financial security in your later years. Integrating these essential tools into your broader planning strategy is not just advisable but crucial for ensuring a secure and peace-filled future for you and your family.

Talking to Family About Senior Living Options

♥

Opening the Dialogue

1. **Choose the Right Time and Place**: Opt for a setting where everyone feels comfortable and can speak freely. Avoid times when family members are stressed, rushed, or distracted.

2. **Be Prepared**: Research the options beforehand so you can provide concrete information. Have some printed material or web resources available to share.

3. **Be Inclusive**: Involve all relevant family members and the senior(s) in question to ensure that everyone has a say.

4. **Start Gently**: This is a sensitive subject. Open the conversa-

tion in a non-threatening way, perhaps by discussing a recent event that makes this topic relevant.

Addressing Concerns

1. **Listen First**: Before you share your views, ask for theirs. Understanding their concerns and opinions will make them more likely to listen to you in return.

2. **Address Emotional Issues**: The prospect of aging and possibly losing independence can be scary. Acknowledge these feelings without judgment.

3. **Be Clear About Financial Realities**: Money is often a significant concern. Be upfront about costs and discuss how they will be managed.

4. **Talk About Medical Needs**: Be prepared to discuss current and possible future medical issues that might make different living situations more or less suitable.

How to Deal with Resistance

1. **Be Patient**: Accept that you may need multiple conversations to arrive at a decision.

2. **Seek Professional Guidance**: Sometimes it helps to have a neutral third party, like a counselor or medical professional, facilitate the discussion.

3. **Provide Examples**: Share stories or information about other people who have successfully made a similar transition.

4. **Address Fears Directly**: If the senior is concerned about losing their independence, discuss how modern senior living options often provide more freedom, not less.

5. **Test the Waters**: Suggest trying the new living arrangement on a temporary basis, which may make the decision feel less daunting.

Conclusion

Talking to family about senior living options is often a difficult but necessary conversation. Planning and patience are key. It's essential to approach the discussion with openness, empathy, and a willingness to consider everyone's point of view. Being prepared and understanding the different facets—from emotional and health needs to financial capabilities—can make the process smoother and more productive for everyone involved.

Medicare, Medicaid, and Insurance in the US and Canada

♥

Introduction

When planning for senior living in the US and Canada, it's essential to understand the different healthcare and insurance options available. While the two countries have some similarities in healthcare provision, their systems are fundamentally different. In the US, healthcare is primarily private, supplemented by Medicare and Medicaid for specific populations. Canada offers universal healthcare, covered mainly by provincial plans.

United States

Medicare

- **What it Covers**: Primarily for seniors aged 65 and older, it has different parts covering hospitalization (Part A), outpatient services (Part B), and prescription drugs (Part D).

- **When to Apply**: Initial enrollment begins three months before the individual turns 65 and extends three months after the 65th birthday.

- **Senior Living Impact**: Medicare doesn't typically cover long-term residential care but may cover limited stays in skilled nursing facilities or rehabilitation centers.

Medicaid

- **What it Covers**: Healthcare for low-income individuals, including some seniors. Coverage varies by state.

- **Eligibility**: Based on income and assets.

- **Senior Living Impact**: Medicaid can cover some long-term care costs, depending on the state's specific rules.

Canada

Provincial Health Plans

- **What it Covers**: Varies by province but generally includes hospital stays and doctor visits.

- **Eligibility**: Usually based on residency in a specific province.

- **Senior Living Impact**: Long-term care facilities may be partially covered, but additional insurance or out-of-pocket payment is often needed for private or semi-private rooms.

Private Insurance

- **Types**: Supplemental plans can cover what provincial plans don't, such as prescription drugs and specialized therapies.

- **Considerations**: Usually an out-of-pocket cost and coverage varies.

Private Insurance (Both Countries)

- **Types**. Long term care insurance, supplemental health plans, etc.

- **Considerations**: Policies can widely vary, and it's essential to understand what is and is not covered.

How These Options Affect Living Choices

- **Aging in Place**: In the US, Medicare and private insurance may cover some home modifications. In Canada, provincial plans are less likely to cover these costs.

- **Assisted Living and Nursing Homes**: In the US, Medicaid and long-term care insurance can help. In Canada, provincial plans may cover basic care in long-term facilities, but additional private insurance is often advisable.

- **Specialized Care Units**: Medicaid in the US and private insurance in Canada may help offset the high costs of specialized units like memory care.

Conclusion

Whether in the US or Canada, understanding the complexities of Medicare, Medicaid, and insurance options is crucial for making informed decisions about senior living. Each country has its own set of benefits and limitations, and a thorough understanding of these, possibly in consultation with a financial advisor, is crucial for future planning.

Medical Insurances for Senior Living in the US and Canada

♥

Medicare

- **What it Covers**: Medicare primarily covers seniors aged 65 and older and provides different types of coverage: Part A (Hospital Insurance), Part B (Medical Insurance), Part C (Medicare Advantage Plans), and Part D (Prescription Drug Plans).

- **When to Apply**: The initial enrollment period for Medicare starts three months before turning 65 and ends three months after the 65th birthday.

- **Senior Living Impact**: Medicare typically does not cover long-term care costs like assisted living or nursing homes but may cover certain aspects like rehabilitation services and skilled nursing care for a limited time.

Medicaid

- **What it Covers**: Medicaid provides healthcare coverage to low-income individuals and may cover costs that Medicare does not, including some long-term care options.

- **Eligibility**: Varies by state, but generally based on income and assets.

- **Senior Living Impact**: Medicaid can sometimes cover the costs of certain long-term care facilities, depending on the state and individual circumstances.

Private Insurance

- **Types**: Beyond government programs, there are private insurance options like long-term care insurance, supplemental health insurance, and life insurance policies that can be converted to senior care payments.

- **Considerations**: Policies and coverage can vary widely. It's essential to read the fine print and consult a financial advisor.

How These Options Affect Living Choices

- **Aging in Place**: Medicare and private insurance may cover some home health care costs or modifications needed to age in place.

- **Assisted Living and Nursing Homes**: Medicaid and long-term care insurance are more likely to help with these costs. Medicare will generally not cover them unless under specific, short-term conditions.

- **Specialized Care Units**: Medicaid and private insurance can sometimes offset the high costs of specialized care, such as memory care units.

Conclusion

Navigating the maze of Medicare, Medicaid, and insurance options can be challenging but is vital for making informed decisions about senior living. DependingDifferent financial tools can be more or less applicable depending on your choice—whether aging in place, moving to an assisted living facility, or requiring specialized care, understanding of these options, possibly in consultation with a financial advisor, can be invaluable in planning a secure, comfortable future.

Tax Benefits and Penalties for Senior Living in the US and Canada

♥

United States

Benefits:

1. **Medical Expense Deductions**: Seniors can deduct qualified medical expenses that exceed 7.5% of their adjusted gross income. This can include some long-term care costs and home modifications for medical reasons.

2. **Selling the Home**: Individuals over 65 may be able to exclude up to $250,000 ($500,000 for couples) of gain from the sale of their primary residence, provided certain conditions are met.

3. **Retirement Account Withdrawals**: Some accounts, like Roth IRAs, offer tax-free withdrawals for seniors.

4. **Social Security Benefits**: A portion may be tax-free depending on your total income and filing status.

Penalties:

1. **Early Withdrawal**: Taking money out of retirement accounts before age 59½ usually incurs a penalty.

2. **Required Minimum Distributions (RMDs)**: Failure to withdraw the RMD from certain retirement accounts after age 72 can result in significant penalties.

Canada

Benefits:

1. **Age Amount Tax Credit**: Seniors may qualify for a non-refundable tax credit if they are 65 or older by the end of the tax year.

2. **Pension Income Splitting**: Up to 50% of eligible pension

income can be split with a spouse to reduce the overall tax burden.

3. **Medical Expenses**: Like in the US, some medical expenses can be claimed as a non-refundable tax credit, including some long-term care costs.

4. **Disability Tax Credit**: If a senior is significantly restricted in daily activities, they may qualify for this non-refundable tax credit.

Penalties:

1. **Old Age Security (OAS) Clawback**: If your income exceeds a certain threshold, you may have to repay part or all of your OAS pension.

2. **RRSP Over-Contribution**: Over-contributing to a Registered Retirement Savings Plan can result in penalties.

Implications for Senior Living Choices:

- **Aging in Place**: Tax benefits in both countries may help offset the cost of making the home safer or more accessible.

- **Assisted Living/Nursing Home**: In both the US and Canada, some costs associated with assisted living or nursing homes may be deductible under medical expenses.

- **Specialized Care Units**: The higher costs associated with these may qualify for medical expense deductions, but you should consult a tax advisor for specifics.

Conclusion

Understanding the tax benefits and penalties associated with aging can help seniors and their families make more informed decisions about their living arrangements. Given the complexity of tax laws in both the US and Canada, consulting a tax advisor is highly advisable for tailored advice.

Independence and Autonomy in Senior Living

♥

The Importance of Maintaining Independence

1. **Psychological Well-being**: A sense of independence is linked to better mental health, including lower rates of depression and higher self-esteem.

2. **Physical Health**: Maintaining an independent lifestyle often encourages physical activity and regular routines, contributing to better overall health.

3. **Quality of Life**: Being able to make choices about one's daily activities increases satisfaction and contributes to a more fulfilling life.

4. **Social Engagement**: Independence often allows seniors to maintain social networks, providing emotional support and reducing feelings of isolation.

5. **Cognitive Function**: Regular activities and social interactions that independence allows can help keep the mind sharp.

Strategies for Staying Autonomous

1. **Stay Physically Active**: Exercise regularly to maintain muscle mass and cardiovascular health, which will help in performing day-to-day activities independently.

2. **Utilize Technology**: From smartphone apps that remind you to take medication to emergency response systems, technology can assist in maintaining independence.

3. **Adapt the Home**: Simple modifications like grab bars in the bathroom, better lighting, and anti-slip flooring can make a home safer and more navigable, thereby promoting independence.

4. **Stay Socially Connected**: Maintain and develop your social network. Strong social ties are associated with better cognitive function and emotional well-being.

5. **Continued Learning**: Keep the brain active by learning new skills, taking up hobbies, or even going back to school.

6. **Consult Professionals**: Engage with healthcare providers,

occupational therapists, and perhaps financial advisors to create a strategy for maintaining autonomy.

7. **Financial Independence**: Budget carefully to ensure that financial constraints do not limit your options and autonomy.

8. **Be Proactive About Health**: Regular check-ups and screenings can catch health problems before they become debilitating. Following a nutritious diet and taking prescribed medications can also help in maintaining independence.

Conclusion

Maintaining independence and autonomy as one ages is crucial for a variety of reasons, from emotional well-being to physical health. While challenges can arise, there are numerous strategies, both behavioral and technological, to help seniors live a more independent and fulfilling life. The key is to start planning early and to make adjustments as needed, so the golden years can be spent in a way that aligns with one's values and desires.

Making the

Transition

♥

Planning the Move

Planning the move to a senior living facility or making modifications to age in place is a process that requires thoughtful preparation. The planning stage should ideally involve not just the senior, but also family members, caregivers, and possibly even healthcare providers. Address key questions like:

- What kind of living arrangement best suits the individual's current and projected health status?

- What is the financial scope for the move?

- Which facilities have the amenities and services that align with the individual's needs and lifestyle?

Create a timeline that breaks down all steps leading up to the move, including when to begin decluttering, when to visit potential new homes, and when to start the actual moving process. A well-laid-out plan will make the transition smoother for everyone involved.

Emotional Preparation

Moving to a new living environment or making significant changes to the current one can be emotionally taxing for seniors and their families. It's crucial to acknowledge and address these emotions early on. Discuss any fears, expectations, and hopes openly. Involve the senior in the decision-making process as much as possible to help them feel empowered and respected. Be sensitive to signs of stress or apprehension, and consider seeking the counsel of a mental health professional if needed.

Practical Tips

1. **Downsizing:** Consider what belongings will be needed in the new living situation and what can be sold, donated, or given to family members.

2. **Visit in Advance:** If moving to a facility, visit multiple times at different times of day to get a feel for the environment.

3. **Financials:** Make sure all financial paperwork is in order, including understanding the billing cycle at the new residence and any financial aid that might be available.

4. **Healthcare Transition:** Ensure a seamless transition of medical records, prescription medicines, and any ongoing treatments.

5. **Home Setup:** Whether aging in place with modifications or moving to a facility, ensure that the living space is set up for convenience, safety, and comfort before the move.

6. **Emergency Contacts:** Keep a list of all important contacts handy, and share them with the facility's staff and family members.

The transition to a new phase of senior living can be challenging, but thorough planning, emotional preparation, and practical considerations can significantly ease the process for the senior and their family.

Resources and Tools

♥

Checklists

1. **Senior Living Options Checklist**: This checklist could cover amenities, healthcare services, financial considerations, and legal prerequisites for each living option considered.

2. **Medical Needs Checklist**: Use this to assess the level of medical care required, whether it's basic assistance with daily activities or more intensive care for chronic conditions.

3. **Financial Checklist**: Cover all income sources, assets, liabilities, and expected future expenses. Include potential sources of financial aid, such as government programs or family contributions.

4. **Legal Checklist**: This should encompass all legal documents needed, such as a will, power of attorney, and healthcare directives.

5. **Emotional and Social Needs Checklist**: List factors like

proximity to family and friends, available social activities, and emotional support systems.

Financial Planning Tools

1. **Budget Planners**: Many online tools and apps can help create a budget for senior living expenses.

2. **Cost Calculators**: These can compare the costs of aging in place, independent living, assisted living, and nursing homes.

3. **Retirement Savings Calculators**: These tools can provide an overview of how long your retirement savings may last under different scenarios.

4. **Medicare/Medicaid Eligibility Tools**: Online questionnaires can help determine eligibility for government aid programs in the U.S.

Directory of Services and Communities

1. **Local and State Directories**: Government websites often list accredited senior living communities and services.

2. **Websites and Apps**: Several websites and apps specialize in providing comprehensive directories of senior living options, complete with reviews and ratings.

3. **Healthcare Provider Network Directories**: These can be useful for finding facilities and services covered under your insurance plan.

4. **Community Centers and Libraries**: These often provide free resources, including directories and sometimes even personal advisors who can guide you through the selection process.

5. **Specialized Directories for Memory Care, Rehabilitation, or Hospice**: These can be particularly useful for finding facilities geared towards specialized care needs.

6. **Veterans Directories**: For veterans, specific directories list facilities and services that may offer special accommodations or financial aid.

By utilizing these checklists, financial planning tools, and directories, individuals and families can make more informed and tailored choices regarding senior living options. Each of these resources contributes to a more holistic approach to planning for this significant life change.

Senior Living Options Checklist Template

General Information

- Name of Facility/Option: ______________________________

- Location: ______________________________

- Contact Information: ______________________________

- Website: ______________________________

Amenities

- Dining Services

- Fitness Center

- Recreational Activities

- Transportation Services

- Outdoor Spaces (gardens, patios, etc.)

- Pet-Friendly

- Internet/Wi-Fi

- Other: _______________________

Healthcare Services

- 24/7 Medical Staff

- Medication Management

- Physical Therapy

- Memory Care Unit

- Routine Check-ups

- Emergency Response System

- Other: _______________________

Financial Considerations

- Monthly Cost: _______________________

- Application Fee: _______________________

- Security Deposit: _______________________

- Inclusions in Monthly Fee (utilities, meals, etc.)

- Extra Costs (additional amenities, services)

- Payment Options: _______________________

- Financial Aid or Subsidies Available

Legal Prerequisites

- Lease Terms

- Termination Policy

- Insurance Requirements

- Visitor Policy

- Other Legal Documents Required: _______________________

Emotional and Social Factors

- Proximity to Family: _______________________

- Social Activities Available: _______________________

- Community Engagement: _______________________

- Spiritual   or   Religious   Services: _______________________

- Other: _______________________

Safety and Accessibility

- Security Measures (guards, cameras, etc.)

- Handrails and Ramps

- Elevators

- Emergency Exits

- Other: _______________________

Additional Notes

-

-

-

Medical Needs Checklist Template for Senior Living Options

❤️

Personal Information

- Name: ____________________________

- Date of Birth: ____________________________

- Address: ____________________________

- Emergency Contact: ____________________________

- Contact Information for Emergency Contact:

____

Medical History

- List of Chronic Conditions: _______________________________

- Previous Surgeries and Dates: _______________________________

- Allergies: _______________________________

- Current Medications and Dosages: _______________________________

Primary Care

- Primary Physician: _______________________________

- Physician's Contact Information: _______________________________

- Date of Last Check-up: _______________________________

Specialized Care Needs

- Need for Memory Care: Yes / No

- Physical Therapy Needs: Yes / No

- Occupational Therapy Needs: Yes / No

- Speech Therapy Needs: Yes / No

Mobility

- Able to move without assistance: Yes / No

- Requires walker or wheelchair: Yes / No

- Needs help with transfers (bed to chair etc.): Yes / No

Daily Living Activities

- Needs assistance with feeding: Yes / No

- Needs assistance with bathing: Yes / No

- Needs assistance with dressing: Yes / No

- Needs assistance with toileting: Yes / No

Sensory Needs

- Visual impairments: Yes / No

- Hearing impairments: Yes / No

- Other sensory issues: ________________________________

Mental Health

- Diagnosed mental health conditions: _______________________

- Current mental health medications: _______________________

Financial and Insurance Information

- Health Insurance Provider: _______________________

- Policy Number: _______________________

- Coverage limitations or exclusions: _______________________

Miscellaneous

- Dietary Restrictions: _______________________

- Preferred Pharmacy: _______________________

- Current Social Activities / Clubs / Groups: _______________________

End-of-Life Preferences

- Do Not Resuscitate Order (DNR): Yes / No

- Living Will: Yes / No

- Power of Attorney for Health Care: Yes / No

This comprehensive checklist is meant to provide a full picture of the medical needs that should be considered when evaluating senior living options. It is advisable to consult healthcare providers and consider this information alongside other factors like costs, amenities, and location.

Financial Checklist Template for Senior Living Options

♥

Personal Information

- Name: _______________________________

- Date of Birth: _______________________________

- Address: _______________________________

- Emergency Contact: _______________________________

- Contact Information for Emergency Contact: _______________________________

Income Sources

- Social Security: ___________________________________

- Pensions: ___________________________________

- Annuities: ___________________________________

- Investments: ___________________________________

- Rental Income: ___________________________________

- Other Income Sources: ___________________________________

Monthly Expenses

- Rent/Mortgage: ___________________________________

- Utilities: ___________________________________

- Food: ___________________________________

- Transportation: ___________________________________

- Healthcare: ___________________________________

- Insurance Premiums: ___________________________________

- Other Expenses: ___________________________________

Savings and Investments

- Checking Account Balance:

____

- Savings   Account   Balance:

____

- Retirement Funds: _________________________________

- Stocks and Bonds: _________________________________

- Real Estate: _________________________________

- Other Investments: _________________________________

Insurance Information

- Health   Insurance   Provider:

____

- Life   Insurance   Provider:

____

- Long-term   Care   Insurance   Provider:

____

- Policy Numbers: _________________________________

Legal Documents

- Will: Yes / No

- Power of Attorney: Yes / No

- Living Will: Yes / No

- Trusts: _______________________________

Debts

- Mortgage: _______________________________

- Car Loans: _______________________________

- Credit Card Debts: _______________________________

- Student Loans: _______________________________

- Medical Bills: _______________________________

- Other Debts: _______________________________

Tax Considerations

- Last Tax Return Filed for Year:
  ____

- Deductions or Credits You Qualify For:
  ____

Budget for Senior Living

- Estimated Cost of Desired Senior Living Option:
  ____

- Additional Costs (e.g., entrance fees, amenities):

  ____

Miscellaneous

- Financial Advisor: _______________________________

- Advisor's Contact Information:

  ____

This comprehensive financial checklist aims to provide a full overview of the financial aspects to consider when evaluating senior living options. Consult with a financial advisor to ensure that you're making a decision that aligns with your financial capabilities and goals.

Emotional and Social Needs Checklist for Senior Living Options

♥

E motional Well-being

- Emotional Resilience

  - Can manage day-to-day emotional challenges: Yes / No

  - Requires emotional support: Yes / No

- Mental Health

  - Undergoing mental health treatment: Yes / No

  - Needs regular emotional check-ins: Yes / No

- Sense of Purpose

  - Engages in activities that bring joy and purpose: Yes / No

  - Needs assistance in finding purposeful activities: Yes / No

- Social Support

- Family Support

  - Frequency of visits: _______________________________

  - Availability for emotional support: High / Medium / Low

- Friendships

  - Number of close friends: _______________________

  - Frequency of social interactions: High / Medium / Low

- Community Involvement

  - Regularly participates in community events: Yes / No

  - Wants to be more involved in the community: Yes / No

- Recreational Needs

- Hobbies and Interests

  - List current hobbies: _______________________

- ○ Interested in learning new hobbies: Yes / No

- Exercise and Physical Activity

  - ○ Currently exercises: Yes / No

  - ○ Preferred   types   of   exercise:
    ____

- Social Activities

  - ○ Enjoys group activities: Yes / No

  - ○ Types   of   preferred   social   activities:
    ____

- Compatibility with Living Options

- Independent Living

  - ○ Emotional and social needs met: Yes / No

- Assisted Living

  - ○ Emotional and social needs met: Yes / No

- Nursing Home

  - ○ Emotional and social needs met: Yes / No

- Other specialized facilities

  - ○ Emotional and social needs met: Yes / No

- Miscellaneous

- Preferred   Communication   Method: _______________________

- Any   Special   Social   or   Emotional   Needs: _______________________

This checklist aims to assess the emotional and social needs crucial for selecting an appropriate senior living option. It is essential to consult with healthcare professionals, therapists, and social workers for a more thorough evaluation.

Legal Checklist for Senior Living Options

Personal Information

- Full Name: _______________________________

- Date of Birth: _______________________________

- Current Address: _______________________________

- Social Security Number: _______________________________

- Emergency Contact: _______________________________

Estate Planning Documents

- Last willt

    ○ Created: Yes / No

    ○ Last Updated: ___________________________

- Trusts

    ○ Created: Yes / No

    ○ Types of Trusts: ___________________________

    ○ Last Updated: ___________________________

- Living Will

    ○ Created: Yes / No

    ○ Last Updated: ___________________________

Power of Attorney

- Financial Power of Attorney

    ○ Created: Yes / No

    ○ Agent's Name: ___________________________

    ○ Last Updated: ___________________________

- Medical Power of Attorney

    ○ Created: Yes / No

- ○ Agent's Name: _______________________________

- ○ Last Updated: _______________________________

Healthcare Documents

- HIPAA Release Form

  - ○ Created: Yes / No

  - ○ Last Updated: _______________________________

- Advanced Healthcare Directive

  - ○ Created: Yes / No

  - ○ Last Updated: _______________________________

- DNR (Do Not Resuscitate) Order

  - ○ Created: Yes / No

Guardianship and Conservatorship

- Legal Guardian (if applicable)

  - ○ Name: _______________________________

  - ○ Relationship: _______________________________

- Conservator (if applicable)

  - ○ Name: _______________________________

    ○ Relationship: _______________________________

Financial Planning Documents

- Retirement Plans and Pensions

  ○ Details: _______________________________

- Investment Accounts

  ○ Details: _______________________________

Contracts and Agreements

- Lease Agreements

  ○ Details: _______________________________

- Business Agreements

  ○ Details: _______________________________

Miscellaneous

- Attorney Contact Information:

  ____

- Important Legal Dates: _______________________________

This comprehensive legal checklist is intended to cover a wide range of legal aspects related to senior living. It's crucial to consult legal advisors to ensure all documents are updated, accurate, and aligned with current laws and personal wishes.

Case Studies

♥

Case Study 1: Aging in Place

Problem: Mr. Johnson, a 75-year-old widower, wants to stay in his long-time home but struggles with mobility.

Solution: A comprehensive home assessment was conducted to identify safety risks. Grab bars were installed in the bathroom, a stair-lift was added, and a personal emergency response system was set up. Regular in-home care services were also arranged for housekeeping and medication management assistance.

Outcome: Mr. Johnson could safely continue living in his home, preserving his independence while ensuring his well-being.

Case Study 2: Assisted Living

Problem: Mrs. Smith, 82, had begun to forget to take her medications and was neglecting her hygiene.

Solution: After discussing the options, her family decided on an assisted living community specializing in mild cognitive issues and medication management.

Outcome: Mrs. Smith moved into her new community, where she receives regular assistance with medication and daily activities, enhancing her quality of life.

Case Study 3: Nursing Home

Problem: Mr. Patel, 89, had a severe stroke that left him unable to independently manage daily activities or medical needs.

Solution: After consulting with healthcare providers, the family decided a nursing home was the best option. They selected a facility experienced in stroke rehabilitation and long-term medical care.

Outcome: Mr. Patel receives the 24/7 medical care and rehabilitative services he needs while his family is reassured of his safety and well-being.

Case Study 4: Memory Care Unit

Problem: Ms. Kim, 78, was diagnosed with advanced Alzheimer's and was becoming increasingly disoriented and anxious in her home.

Solution: Her family chose a memory care unit specializing in Alzheimer's and dementia care.

Outcome: In the specialized setting, Ms. Kim receives the individualized care she needs, including activities designed for her cognitive abilities. The family has peace of mind knowing she is safe and cared for.

Case Study 5: Hospice Care

Problem: Mrs. Rodriguez, 93, has terminal cancer and wishes to spend her remaining time comfortably without aggressive treatments.

Solution: Her family and healthcare team decided hospice care was the best option. They chose an in-home hospice care service to allow Mrs. Rodriguez to stay in her home.

Outcome: Mrs. Rodriguez receives compassionate end-of-life care focused on comfort and dignity. Her symptoms are managed effectively, and her family receives emotional support.

Case Study 6: Independent Living

Problem: Mr. and Mrs. Anderson, both in their 70s, found it increasingly challenging to maintain their large family home.

Solution: They decided to downsize and move into an independent living community, where they could enjoy a more manageable living space and access various amenities.

Outcome: The Andersons now reside in a vibrant community where they participate in social activities and no longer worry about home maintenance.

Case Study 7: Rehabilitation Center

Problem: Mrs. Carter, 68, suffered a severe hip fracture and required intensive rehabilitation after her surgery.

Solution: Her healthcare team recommended a rehabilitation center where she could receive specialized physical therapy and nursing care.

Outcome: After weeks of dedicated therapy, Mrs. Carter regained her mobility and could return home, thanks to the support she received at the rehabilitation center.

Case Study 8: Specialized Care Facility - Parkinson's Disease

Problem: Mr. Davis, 81, had advanced Parkinson's disease and needed comprehensive care tailored to his condition.

Solution: His family chose a specialized care facility with expertise in Parkinson's care, providing him with a structured environment and specialized therapies.

Outcome: Mr. Davis experienced significant improvements in his symptoms, and his family was relieved to see him thriving in a supportive environment.

Case Study 9: Memory Care Unit (Frontotemporal Dementia)

Problem: Ms. Turner, 70, was diagnosed with frontotemporal dementia, which required specialized care and support.

Solution: Her family selected a memory care unit specializing in frontotemporal dementia, ensuring her unique needs were met.

Outcome: In this specialized unit, Ms. Turner receives personalized care, and her family has peace of mind knowing that her condition is managed with expertise.

Case Study 10: Combination of Aging in Place and In-Home Care

Problem: Mr. White, 87, wished to continue living in his home but needed assistance with certain daily activities.

Solution: His family decided to combine aging in place with in-home care services, providing him with the support he needed while staying in his familiar environment.

Outcome: Mr. White enjoys the comfort of his home and receives the necessary assistance to maintain his independence and quality of life.

These case studies offer a glimpse into the diverse scenarios seniors and their families may face. Understanding that every case is unique and multiple resources should be consulted in making decisions.

Expert Opinions on Senior Living Options

♥

To provide valuable insights, I've gathered opinions from healthcare providers, gerontologists, and other professionals in the field of senior care. Here are their thoughts on various senior living options:

Dr. Sarah Mitchell, Gerontologist

On Aging in Place: "Aging in place can be a great option for seniors who value familiarity. However, it's essential to assess home safety and consider the availability of support services to ensure a safe and comfortable environment."

On Assisted Living: "Assisted living can provide the right balance of independence and support. It's crucial to choose a facility that offers tailored care plans to meet the individual's specific needs."

On Memory Care Units: "Memory care units are designed to cater to the unique challenges of dementia and Alzheimer's. Specialized care, secure environments, and sensory-focused activities can significantly improve the quality of life for residents."

Dr. Robert Johnson, Family Physician

On Nursing Homes: "Nursing homes are ideal for individuals with complex medical needs. They offer 24/7 care, but it's important for families to stay involved in their loved one's care and monitor their well-being."

On Hospice Care: "Hospice care emphasizes comfort and dignity at the end of life. It's a compassionate choice for those with terminal illnesses, providing physical, emotional, and spiritual support."

On Independent Living Communities: "Independent living communities promote an active and social lifestyle. Seniors enjoy the freedom of private apartments while having access to amenities and social activities."

Emily Davis, Senior Care Coordinator

On Financial Planning: "Seniors and their families should start financial planning early. Consider long-term care insurance, Medicaid eligibility, and seek professional advice to ensure you're financially prepared for senior living."

On Emotional Needs: "Emotional well-being is often overlooked but crucial. Regular social interactions, engaging activities, and emotional support are essential for a senior's overall happiness."

On Legal Planning: "Establishing a Power of Attorney and creating a comprehensive estate plan can provide peace of mind and ensure that your wishes are honored in case you can't make decisions independently."

These expert opinions underscore the importance of a holistic approach when considering senior living options. Each individual's unique needs and circumstances should guide the decision-making process, with careful consideration of medical, financial, emotional, and legal aspects.

Appendix

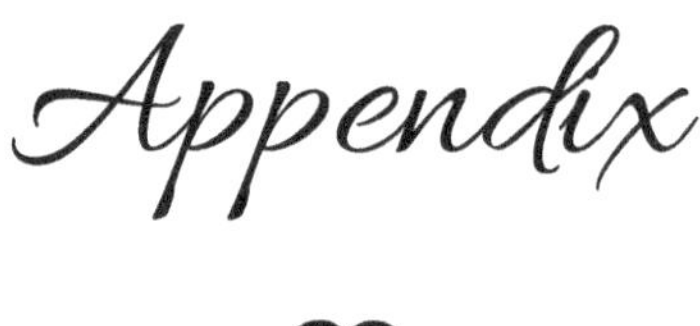

Glossary of Terms

1. **Aging in Place**: The practice of staying in one's own home as one grows older, rather than moving to a senior-specific living arrangement.

2. **Assisted Living**: A residential option for seniors who need assistance with some daily activities such as bathing, dressing, and medication management.

3. **Independent Living**: A residential living setting for elderly or senior adults that may or may not provide hospitality or supportive services.

4. **Nursing Home**: A facility for the residential care of elderly people who require constant nursing care and have significant deficiencies with activities of daily living.

5. **Memory Care Unit**: Specialized units within facilities that offer focused care for individuals with memory issues, in-

cluding Alzheimer's and other dementias.

6. **Rehabilitation Centers**: Facilities specialized in providing intensive physical therapy, occupational therapy, and other types of therapy.

7. **Hospice Care**: Specialized care designed to provide comfort and support to patients and their families when a life-limiting illness no longer responds to cure-oriented treatments.

8. **Power of Attorney**: A legal document allowing one person to act on another's behalf for legal or financial issues.

9. **Estate Planning**: The act of preparing for the transfer of a person's wealth and assets after their death.

10. **Medicare/Medicaid**: U.S. government-sponsored healthcare programs, with Medicare primarily serving people over 65 and Medicaid serving low-income individuals.

11. **Socialized Healthcare**: Canadian government-sponsored healthcare, primarily funded through taxes.

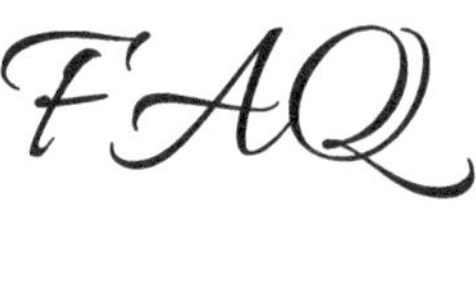

FAQ

Frequently Asked Questions

1. **What is the difference between assisted living and a nursing home?**

- Assisted living provides help with some daily activities but not constant nursing care, while a nursing home provides intensive nursing care and medical treatments.

1. **Does Medicare cover the cost of a nursing home?**

- Medicare may cover some costs, but there are strict guidelines for eligibility. It's important to check specifics in advance.

1. **What is involved in estate planning?**

- Estate planning includes the preparation of wills, trusts, power of attorney, and other legal documentation to manage your estate after your death.

1. **What is a Memory Care Unit?**

- A Memory Care Unit is a specialized environment designed for the care and support of individuals with memory issues such as Alzheimer's disease.

1. **How do I open the dialogue about senior living options with my family?**

- Start by acknowledging the emotional weight of the subject and use open-ended questions to guide the discussion. Involve all relevant family members and make sure everyone has a chance to speak.

1. **What modifications can make aging in place safer?**

- Adding grab bars, stairlifts, and improving lighting are some modifications that can make a home safer for seniors.

1. **What are the financial implications of different senior living options?**

- The costs can vary widely based on the level of care needed, the type of facility, and location. Always consider future financial needs as well as current costs.

1. **How do I deal with resistance when discussing senior living options?**

- Resistance is often rooted in fear or misunderstanding. Address concerns openly, provide information, and consider professional advice if necessary.

By comprehensively addressing these questions and understanding key terms, you are better equipped to make informed decisions about senior living, ensuring that you or your loved one experiences a fulfilling and secure later life.

Conclusion

♥

Choosing the right senior living option is multifaceted beyond medical and financial considerations. It also involves a deep understanding of emotional and social needs, crucial for maintaining a high quality of life in the golden years. Comprehensive checklists for each aspect—from medical and financial to emotional and social—can help streamline decision-making, ensuring that all bases are covered. Incorporating tools like Power of Attorney and estate planning into your strategy can secure a stable and fulfilling future. Therefore, it's not just advisable but imperative to approach this significant life transition with a well-rounded, thoughtful plan that aligns with the needs and desires of the individual and their family.

References

1. **National Institute on Aging (NIA)**: NIA provides valuable information on various aspects of aging and senior living options. (Website: https://www.nia.nih.gov/)

2. **AARP**: AARP offers a wide range of resources and articles on topics related to aging, including senior living choices. (Website: https://www.aarp.org/)

3. **Alzheimer's Association**: For information on memory care and dementia-related topics, the Alzheimer's Association is a reputable source. (Website: https://www.alz.org/)

4. **Medicare.gov**: This official U.S. government website provides information on Medicare and Medicaid, which can be important for understanding the financial aspects of senior care. (Website: https://www.medicare.gov/)

5. **Consulting with Healthcare Professionals**: To get personalized advice and expert opinions, consider consulting with gerontologists, family physicians, elder care attorneys,

or senior care coordinators in your local area.

6. **Government of Canada - Seniors**: The official website provides information on programs and services for seniors, including healthcare, pensions, and housing. (Website: htt ps://www.canada.ca/en.html)

7. **Canadian Association on Gerontology (CAG)**: CAG is a professional organization focused on gerontology and aging research. They provide resources and publications related to aging and senior care. (Website: https://cagacg.ca/)

8. **Alzheimer Society of Canada**: For information on dementia care and memory care options, the Alzheimer Society of Canada is a valuable resource. (Website: https://alzheim er.ca/en/Home)

9. **Canadian Network for the Prevention of Elder Abuse (CNPEA)**: CNPEA offers resources and information to prevent elder abuse and promote the well-being of older adults. (Website: https://cnpea.ca/)

10. **Canada's National Pensioners Federation (NPF)**: NPF focuses on issues related to pensions, income security, and the well-being of seniors. (Website: https://npf-fpn.com/)